How to
Measure Angles
from
Foot Radiographs

D1242047

How to
Measure Angles
from
Foot Radiographs

A PRIMER

Alan E. Oestreich

With illustrations by
Tamar Kahane Oestreich

Springer-Verlag
New York   Berlin   Heidelberg
London   Paris   Tokyo

Alan E. Oestreich, M.D.
Division of Radiology
Children's Hospital Medical Center
Cincinnati, Ohio 45229-2899
USA

Oestreich, Alan E.
  How to measure angles from foot radiographs : a primer : by Alan
E. Oestreich with illustrations by Tamar Kahane Oesteich.
    p.   cm.
  ISBN 0-387-97107-6
  1. Foot—Radiography. 2. Foot—Abnormalities—Diagnosis.
  I. Title.
RC951.0371989
617.5'850757—dc20   89-28539
                                                          CIP

Typeset by Compositors Corporation, Cedar Rapids, Iowa.
Printed and bound by Edwards Brothers, Ann Arbor, Michigan
Printed in the United States of America.

9 8 7 6 5 4 3 2 1

ISBN 0-387-97107-6 Springer-Verlag New York Berlin Heidelberg
ISBN 3-540-97107-6 Springer-Verlag Berlin Heidelberg New York

Preface

Why and Wherefore?

Welcome to our little introductory book! It appears in response to beginning students (i.e., especially general radiology residents) who have sought guidance with the methodology of evaluating positional relationships of the feet from radiographs. Since my stepwise "how to" technique has been well received both in the Show-Me state (at the University of Missouri-Columbia) and here in Ohio, it is offered to you as well.

To simulate my conventional teaching method, the informal text has an interactive flavor, which I hope makes it useful for you. Please don't be offended by a touch of simplified walking-through of material here and there. After all, this is a "primer," not a dignified postgraduate treatise. Comments from readers would of course be appreciated by the author.

The majority of illustrations are the result of the collaboration with my dear colleague Tamar, in which she artistically interpreted representative radiographs for you to my specifications. The guidelines I gave her included line drawing outlines of the most pertinent bones, to which straight lines were added as appropriate. As a result certain bones, for example the fibula and many phalanges, are omitted if they are unlikely to enhance the impact of the illustrations. Often, too, the cuneiforms and cuboid remain undifferentiated as one bony element, or only a few of them are drawn, so that attention remains with the key bones involved.

Why Should Angles Be Measured on Radiographs?

Angles provide a relatively objective indication of positional relationships of bones. Significant abnormalities in such relationships can lead to pain. In the developing child, growth of large and small bones alike may be asymmetrically and increasingly modified for the worse in the face of positional abnormality. Moreover, and indeed more importantly, impairment or overstimulation of all or part of an enchondral growth plate (or other enchondral or membranous growth region) tends to accelerate asymmetry during growth and development.

Measurement of angles, then, permits recognition and documentation of significant abnormality of bones and joints that may benefit from orthopedic evaluation and treatment, as well as a means of evaluating the effectiveness of such treatment. In real life, positioning the foot and other body parts for radiographs is fraught with potential pitfalls, beyond the scope of this book. Our purpose instead is to provide a useful introduction into the methodology of measuring angles on radiographs that have been obtained, in order to provide the orthopedist, podiatrist, or other health care professional with **useful** information relevant to the possible care of her/his patient.

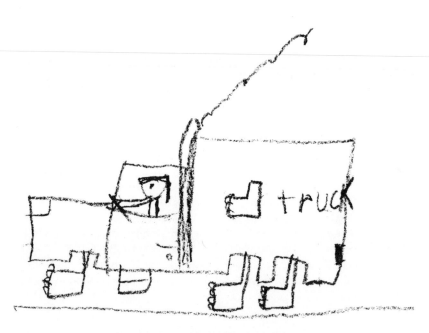

"Foot Truck" by Michael P. Oestreich, age 6.

Acknowledgments

Our thanks to Carol Amundsen for her skilled assistance with manuscript typing, revision, and correction. We are grateful to Bernhard Lewerich and James Costello of the Springer-Verlag for their interest, encouragement, and willingness to support new ideas. Thanks are also due to Dr. Mike Ozonoff and Saunders for permission to excerpt some of his artwork from *Pediatric Orthopedic Radiology,* to the *Journal of Bone and Joint Surgery* for permission to reproduce diagrams and graphs from Dr. VanderWilde's article, and to Thieme-Verlag for permission to reprint several illustrations from the *Atlas of Pediatric Orthopedic Radiology,* which I co-authored with Dr. Alvin Crawford. Several line drawings are based on photographs in that *Atlas* as well.

And to Michael, thanks for being so patient while your parents were engaged in the work on this book.

Contents

1
Varus and Valgus

What Are Varus and Valgus?

1. They are *relationships* between a *distal part* of an extremity to an *adjoining proximal part.*
   (a) Usually *bony* parts are considered, but the definition would hold for cartilaginous structures as well.
   (b) examples: — tibia with-respect-to femur
              — proximal tibia epiphysis
                with-respect-to
                tibia diaphysis
   but not: — radius shaft with-respect-to ulna shaft
2. They are *abnormal positional relations* in the *coronal plane** (i.e., side-to-side plane) considered in *anatomic position* (with regard to pronation, supination, and internal or external rotation, all in neutral); in which the relationship of the distal part to the proximal part are *evaluated as if the proximal part were in its normal anatomic position.*

That's a mouthful, but please check out Figure 1, which illustrates this definition.

3. So they are defined as follows:

   varus: An angulation in which the distal part is directed *closer toward* the midline of the body than normal compared to the proximal part, with the proximal part considered in anatomic position.
   valgus: An angulation in which the distal part is directed *further from* the midline of the body than normal compared to the proximal part, when the proximal part is considered as if it were in anatomic position.

---

*For the foot, however, the axial plane (i.e., horizontal).

Suppose that normal looks
like this.

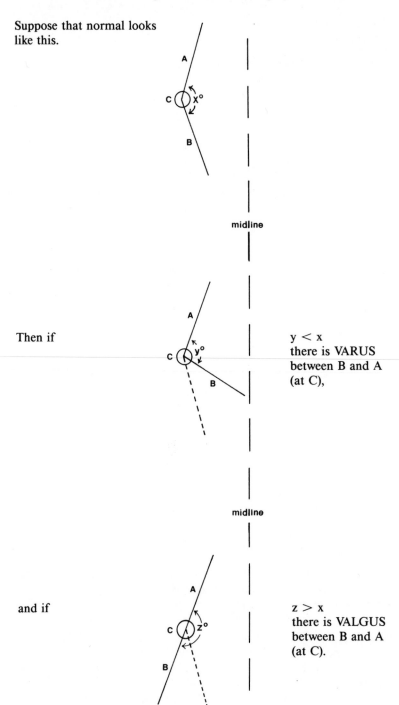

Then if

y < x
there is VARUS
between B and A
(at C),

and if

z > x
there is VALGUS
between B and A
(at C).

FIGURE 1. Varus and valgus illustrated.

Again, suppose that
normal looks like this.

Then if

and if

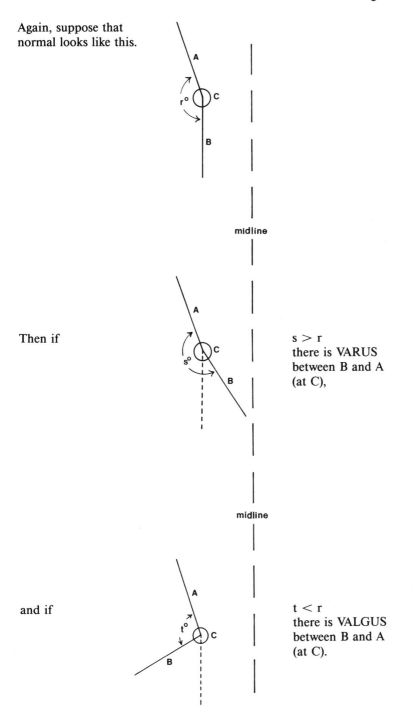

s > r
there is VARUS
between B and A
(at C),

t < r
there is VALGUS
between B and A
(at C).

(In patients with scoliosis, "midline" is taken as an ideal, as if the scoliosis had been completely corrected.) Figure 1 illustrates these definitions abstractly.

In the schematic examples of Figure 1, it has been assumed that the involved parts are positioned so that *the proximal part is in its normal anatomic position* with respect to the midline. This is true in general for evaluation of varus or valgus. For example, in *bow legs* the femur should be considered as if in normal anatomic (i.e., more nearly vertical) position, and the tibia will then be noted to deviate sharply toward the midline and indeed cross it considerably, as in Figure 2.

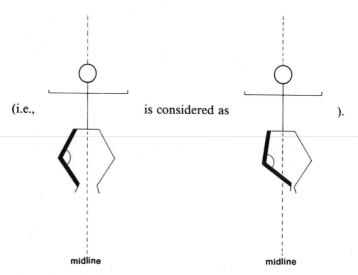

(i.e.,   is considered as   ).

FIGURE 2. Positioning the right femur to its anatomic position in evaluating bow legs.

For purposes of evaluation of varus/valgus, the extremity is also considered in neutral anatomic position with regard to supination and pronation.

Now, let's warm up for the feet by conquering varus and valgus of the *hip.*

Here, by convention we are talking about the relationship of *shaft* to *neck.* At the *hip,* when the angle between the femur neck and the femur shaft is smaller than normal, this is *coxa vara.* When the angle between the neck and the shaft is greater than normal, this is *coxa valga*. (At birth a normal angle may be 150°; in childhood 120° is the lower limit of normal.)

Figure 3 shows how this convention fits into our schema.

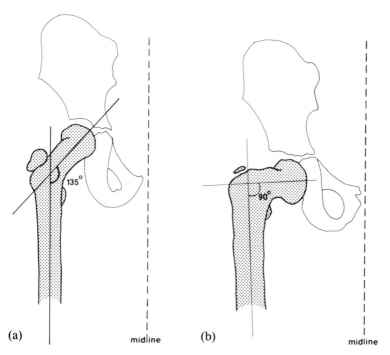

(a)   midline   (b)   midline

FIGURE 3. Relationship of shaft to neck in normal vs. varus hip. (a) Normal hip. (b) Varus hip.

But this angular relationship should be considered as if the proximal part (the femur neck) is in its normal anatomic relation to midline (with the distal part shifting along with it). Figure 4 shows a varus hip with the neck considered as if in normal position. Viewed thus, the distal part (shaft) is clearly deviated *toward* the midline compared to normal.

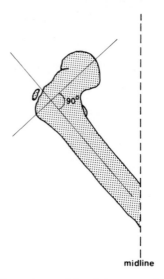

FIGURE 4. Varus hip with neck considered in normal anatomic position.

Now, imagine (or draw) the same kind of line drawings for a valgus relationship at the hip (Figure 5).

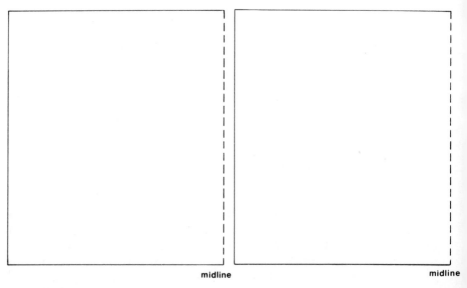

midline   midline

FIGURE 5.

Because of the convention of describing hip varus/valgus according to the neck-shaft angle, there are some hips, such as in achondroplasia, which appear at first varus to the eye, but are relatively valgus by measurement. An example is shown in Figure 6.

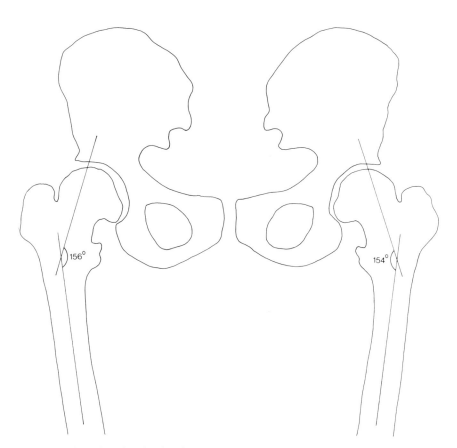

156°   154°

FIGURE 6. Achondroplastic hips.

Now that you have worked out the formal definitions of hip varus and valgus so nicely, let's give you our mnemonic line drawing for these relationships at the *right hip*. The device is to consider the shape of the involved *right* hip as the third letter (in lower case) of the word varus (vara) or valgus (valga) (see Figure 7).

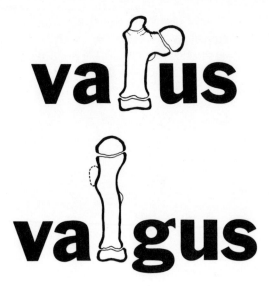

FIGURE 7. Varus/valgus mnemonic. (Reproduced, with permission, from Oestreich AE, Crawford AH. *Atlas of Pediatric Orthopedic Radiology.* Stuttgart: Thieme; 1985:115.)

As we move closer to our region of interest, let's stop briefly at the knee. Here again is the line drawing which fits *knee varus* into our formal definition (see Figure 8).

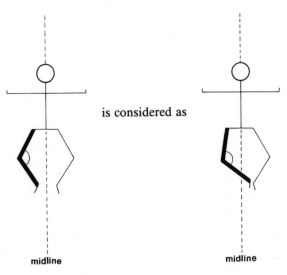

FIGURE 8. Figure 2 repeated.

Again, we invite you to create the equivalent line drawings for knee valgus (Figure 9).

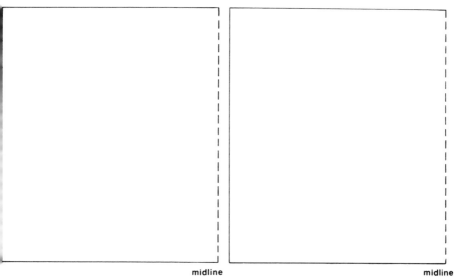

midline   midline

FIGURE 9.

The Germans have helpful lay terms for knee varus and valgus, respectively "O-Bein und X-Bein," which you can translate from the sketches in Figure 10.

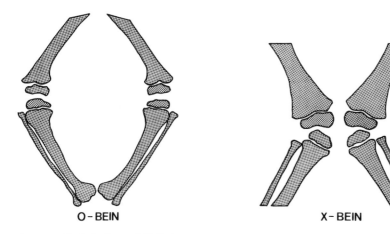

O-BEIN   X-BEIN

FIGURE 10. O-Bein and X-Bein.

In English, the terms "bow legs" and "knock-knees" also get the image across, but less alphabetically. Now, to review, please match the terms from each column:

a. knee varus   C. knock-knees   *e.* O-Bein
b. knee valgus   D. bow legs   *f.* X-Bein

answer: a D *e;* b C *f*

Ending our introductory foray into varus and valgus, let's briefly mention the upper extremity and midbones.

At the elbow, Figure 11 gives an example of **cubitus varus.**

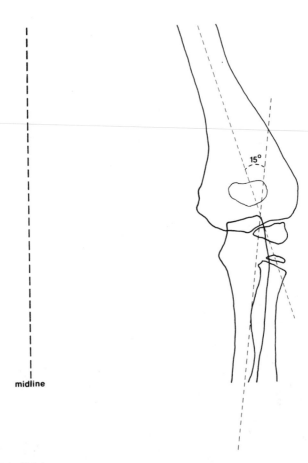

FIGURE 11. Cubitus varus.

In general, *slowing* or cessation of longitudinal (enchondral) *growth* at the *medial* side of a long bone physis would be expected to cause _____ at that site [fill in the blank with valgus or varus, please], because of the continued lateral growth as opposed to impaired medial growth, which imbalance in growth tends to drive the distal part more *medially.* Conversely, slowing at the *lateral side* drives the distal part *laterally,* yielding relative _____ .

On the contrary, *accelerated* enchondral growth at the *medial* side of a physis causes _____ , and at the *lateral* side causes _____ .

snɹɐʌ 'snƃlɐʌ 'snƃlɐʌ 'snɹɐʌ :sɹǝʍsuɐ

Accelerated medial growth may occur, for example, at the proximal tibia physis after a childhood proximal tibia shaft fracture, which often causes proximal tibia valga.

An osteotomy, fracture, or deformity within a bone may similarly be termed varus or valgus if the definition fits (Figure 12).

In each of Figures 12 and 13, the drawing on the left recreates a radiograph, and the drawing on the right considers the same relationship with the proximal part rotated into the vertical.

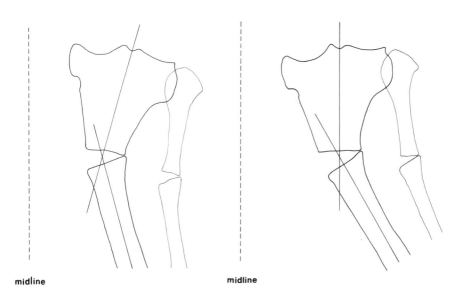

midline   midline

FIGURE 12. Valgus osteotomy (to treat medially tilted ankle, for example).

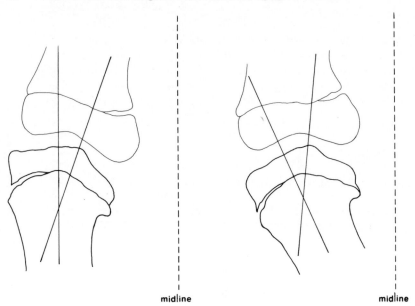

midline   midline

FIGURE 13. Tibia vara (Blount disease—varus between epiphysis and diaphysis).

OK, we're ready for the FOOT!

2
The Hindfoot Frontal View

For a frontal (AP) weightbearing view of a foot, see Figure 14.

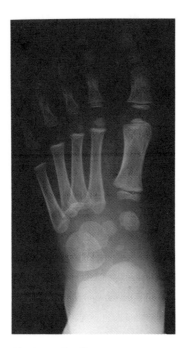

FIGURE 14. Frontal (AP) view of a foot.

1. Please identify the *navicular*, the *talus*, and the *calcaneus*.
2. Which is the most *proximal* bone of the three?
   - navicular?
   - talus?
   - calcaneus?

If you have any doubts, please consult an articulated skeleton or an anatomy textbook, or else look at a lateral film of the hindfoot. Thank you.

Remember, valgus and varus describe the relationship of a distal part to an adjoining proximal part; (except in the case of the forefoot, for which we will make an exception!) Now that we have reestablished which of the talus and calcaneus is more proximal, we are ready to establish the normal angle between them on the frontal *weightbearing* (or simulated weightbearing) film.

A nice round number to remember is a 30° more lateral axis of the calcaneus compared to the talus, measured as in Figure 15.

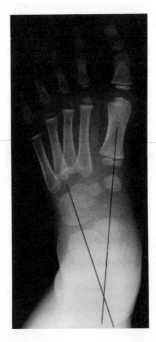

FIGURE 15. Normal talo-calcaneal angle.

It may sometimes be simpler to use the lateral margin of the calcaneus as its axis rather than constructing a midline, especially when the posterior-most calcaneus isn't on the film (Figure 16).

Actually, the frontal talo-calcaneal angle decreases with age during the first decade of life, as nicely charted by Drs. VanderWilde, Staheli, Chew, and Magalon in Figure 17.

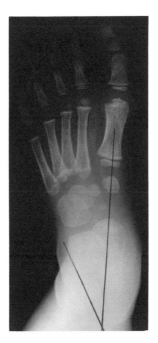

FIGURE 16. Alternate method for calculating the talo-calcaneal angle.

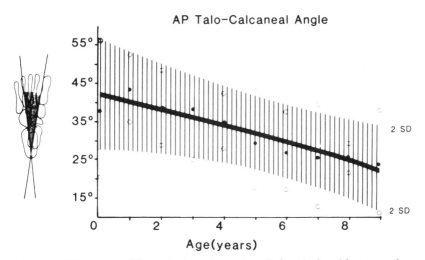

FIGURE 17. Decrease of frontal talo-calcaneal angle in relationship to age during first decade of life. (Reproduced, with permission, from VanderWilde R, Staheli LT, Chew DE, Magalon V. Measurements on radiographs of the foot in normal infants and children. *J Bone Jt Surg.* 1988;70A:407–415.)

So 30° isn't a bad number to remember, if it is recognized that infants have a higher normal value.

Why "weightbearing" or "simulated weightbearing"? you may ask. Because, positional relationships of bones of the lower extremities are most important when bearing weight, especially in consideration of the feet (however, nonweightbearing relationships may have importance at some sites, such as the difficulty in care of the perineum in the severely impaired recumbent child when there is hip valgus and adduction). Moreover, there may be a dramatic difference in foot relationships between weightbearing and not-weightbearing. A foot arch may disappear upon standing in some subjects, for example. And look at the major difference in frontal talo-calcaneal angle in the clinical example given in Figure 18.

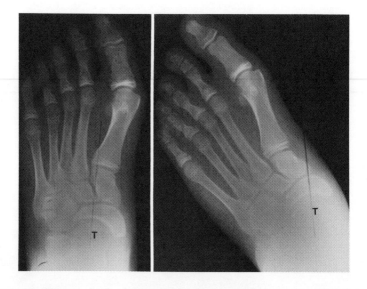

FIGURE 18. Changes in the frontal talo-calcaneal angle between weightbearing and not-weightbearing. The weightbearing foot is shown on your right. (Reproduced, with permission, from Oestreich AE, Crawford AH. *Atlas of Pediatric Orthopedic Radiology.* Stuttgart: Thieme; 1985:114.)

Weightbearing is also more repeatable from one examination to the other (if "wiggly feet" or inconstant positioning doesn't defeat the attempt).

Hindfoot Varus

If the *normal angle* between the *proximal hindfoot bone* (that's the talus, folks) and the distal hindfoot bone (calcaneus) on AP film is about 30°, especially in 6-year-olds, then a significantly *smaller* angle (or negative angle) means that the distal bone is *directed closer to the midline* than it is expected to be. Therefore we have a *varus* relationship.

It doesn't matter where the talus heads when the subject stands—our interest is in the axis of the calcaneus compared with that of the talus. If talus and calcaneus are parallel on the frontal film, the angle is 0°, which is considerably less than 30°, and we have a varus relationship of the hindfoot. It's that straightforward. For example see Figure 19.

Hindfoot Valgus

If the *normal angle* between the *proximal hindfoot bone* (still the talus) and the *distal hindfoot bone* (you know what I mean) on AP film is 30°, especially in 6-year-olds, then a significantly *greater* angle (in the newborn that's above 55° according to Dr. VanderWilde and colleagues) means that the distal bone is *directed further from the midline* than it is expected to be. Therefore we have a *valgus* relationship.

It doesn't matter where the talus heads when the subject stands—our interest is in the axis of the calcaneus compared with that of the talus. If the talus and calcaneus were perpendicular on the frontal film, the angle would be 90°, which is considerably more than 30° (or even than 55° in the newborn), and we would have a valgus relationship of the hindfoot. It's that straightforward. For example see Figure 20.

The *navicular* is actually considered a midfoot bone, but in most children the calcaneus and navicular have a *fixed* relationship to each other, at least in the absence of surgery or deformity. So

if the calcaneal axis is hard to determine,
and
if the navicular is ossified (which it isn't in early life)
and
if you can judge the centering of the navicular (i.e., the concavity of the "boat-bone") on the head of the talus ("ankle bone")
then you get an indirect indication of whether or not the hindfoot is in varus or valgus.

Quite simply, the boat normally should be centered on the talus head (axis of the talus going through the middle of the boat). Compare Figure 21a, b, and c.

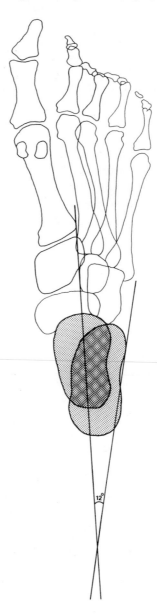

FIGURE 19. Hindfoot varus.

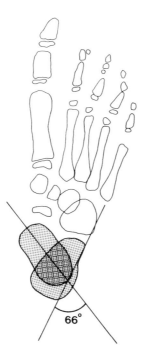

FIGURE 20. Hindfoot valgus.

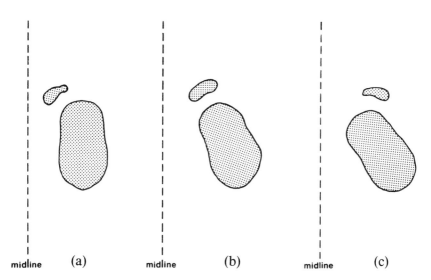

FIGURE 21. Alternative method for calculating hindfoot varus/valgus based on the midfoot relationship of the navicular to the talus. (a) Varus: the boat slips medially. (b) Normal: just fine. (c) Valgus: the boat slips laterally.

Caveats: *Early* navicular ossification may not be central within the cartilaginous model, or it may be multipartite, circumstances which weaken the usefulness of this alternate method. Moreover, any disturbance in the calcaneus-navicular relationship (for example, clubfoot surgery) destroys this method. Finally, "indirect" is not as "direct" as "direct" in evaluating "direction."

Ankle Valgus

Orthopedic experience has demonstrated that hindfoot surgery that addresses foot valgus will not be successful if concommitant **ankle valgus** is not treated as well. In this context, ankle valgus refers to valgus of the *talus* with respect to the *tibia*. Ankle valgus is observed clinically by viewing the weightbearing ankle from behind (the observer may lie prone on the floor with hyperextended neck, or may ask the subject to stand on an elevation in order to make the observer more comfortable). Radiographic evaluation of ankle valgus requires a frontal weightbearing *ankle film,* see Figure 22—foot films are not sufficient.

A talus which is tilted medially or laterally, say in bow legs or knock-knees, is technically not in varus or valgus if its axial axis is in the same direction as that of the longitudinal axis of the tibia.

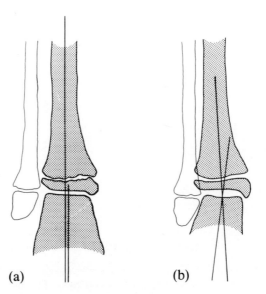

(a)   (b)

FIGURE 22. (a) Normal vs. (b) valgus ankle.

3
The Forefoot Frontal View

The "Talus-First Metatarsal Convention"

At this point we modify one part of the varus/valgus definition worked out earlier—namely the criterion of the adjacent relationship (see page 1).

Whereas, in the unoperated, undeformed foot all the bones of the midfoot and the forefoot tend to maintain a constant relationship to each other and to the calcaneus (more so than to the talus, which is stuck in the ankle mortise),

and, whereas, bones of the midfoot are variably ossified in younger children,

and, whereas, it seems to work pretty well in most cases,

therefore, by convention some observers, myself included, discuss **forefoot varus/valgus** as a relationship between the *talus* and the *first metatarsal,* even though these bones are not truly adjacent (see Figures 23–26). It makes life (during foot evaluation) a lot simpler!

The Normal Forefoot

Put simply, in the normal forefoot *the midline axis of the talus goes through the base of the first metatarsal* on the normal AP weightbearing film.

In more precise terms (if you want them), the midline axis of the talus usually lies a bit lateral to the midline axis of the first metatarsal, but still does cut through the (lateral) base of the first metatarsal.

For still more precise terms, we may consult the chart from Doctors VanderWilde, Staheli, Chew, and Malagon, given in Figure 24.

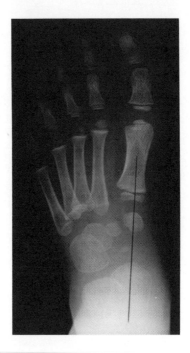

FIGURE 23. Normal talus—first metatarsal relationship. Midline of talus goes through the base of the first metatarsal shaft.

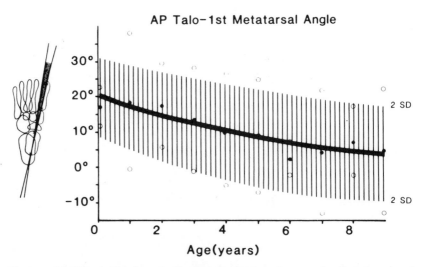

FIGURE 24. Change in the talo-first metatarsal angle over the first decade of life. (Reproduced, with permission, from VanderWilde R, Staheli LT, Chew DE, Magalon V. Measurements on radiographs of the foot in normal infants and children. *J Bone Jt Surg.* 1988;70A:407–415.)

As you see, the axis of the talus approaches the central axis of the first metatarsal more and more during life's first decade.

Now, following the above convention, we are ready to define so-called **forefoot varus.**

(As an aside, if you ignore the foot inversion involved, you may consider the Milton Berle walking posture as forefoot varus. If you haven't observed Uncle Miltie in action, ignore that remark.)

In forefoot varus, *the axis of the distal bone (i.e., the first metatarsal) is directed more medially than normal with respect to the proximal bone* (i.e., the talus).

So, where does the axis of the talus lie at the metatarsal region? It lies _____ to the first metatarsal.

If you said/wrote/thought "medial," you were wrong! It goes lateral, so that the axis of the distal bone lies more medial than the axis of the proximal bone.

Remember, we are talking of the *relative* position of two bones—if the talus axis is directed quite laterally while the first metarsal is straight ahead, it is still forefoot varus. Figure 25 illustrates some forefoot varus.

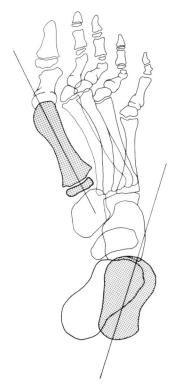

FIGURE 25. Forefoot varus.

And now we are ready to define, using the same convention as above, the so-called **forefoot valgus.**

(As an aside, you may consider the Charlie Chaplin walking posture as forefoot valgus. If you haven't observed the Little Tramp in action, where have you been?)

In forefoot valgus, *the axis of the distal bone (i.e., the first metatarsal) is directed more laterally than normal with respect to the proximal bone* (i.e., the talus).

So, where does the axis of the talus lie at the metatarsal region? It lies _____ to the first metatarsal.

If you said/wrote/thought "lateral," you better go back 2 spaces and review the varus forefoot. It goes medial, so that the axis of the distal bone lies more lateral than the axis of the proximal bone.

Remember, we are talking again of the relative position of two bones—if the talus axis is directed quite medially while the first metatarsal is straight ahead, it is indeed forefoot valgus. Figure 26 illustrates some forefoot valgus.

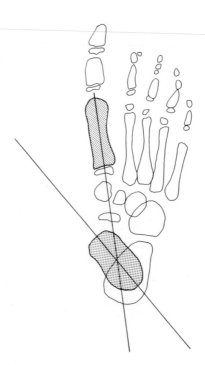

FIGURE 26. Forefoot valgus.

Hallux Valgus, Metatarsus Primus Varus, and Bunionette

Let's apply these techniques for determining varus/valgus to three other relationships of the forefoot.

Best known is hallux valgus. The hallux is the great toe. In **hallux valgus,** the proximal phalanx of the great toe is considered with respect to the first metatarsal.

(proximal part = 1st metatarsal)
(distal part = proximal phalanx of great toe)

Please study Figure 27a and b.

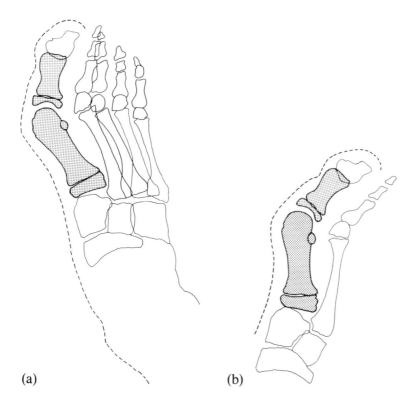

(a)   (b)

FIGURE 27. (a) Hallux valgus. (b) Hallux valgus shown with film rotated to make the metatarsal straight.

This definition does not take into account possible accompanying factors—such as lateral, dorsal, or ventral displacement of the base of the proximal phalanx on the metatarsal head. No, the valgus refers to the relative position of the two bones with respect to each other and to the midline in the axial (horizontal) plane of the foot.

Although the metatarsal is headed medially, it is considered in its anatomic nearly straight position, which makes the axis of the proximal phalanx head quite lateral, as shown in the illustration pair above.

Associated with many cases of hallux valgus, perhaps even a factor in its etiology, is **metatarsus primus varus.** By strict definition, this refers to *a varus relationship of the first metatarsal (distal part) to the medial cuneiform* (proximal part), as in Figure 28.

In everyday practice, the presence and degree of metatarsus primus varus is measured by considering the proximal angle between the first and second metatarsals. If it gets above 10°, that's considered indicative of metatarsus primus varus.

The assumption (or practical guide) is that the second metacarpal axis is a reasonable approximation of the medial cuneiform axis.

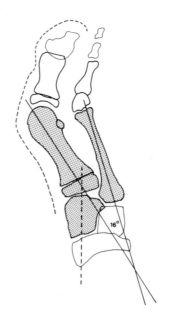

FIGURE 28. Metatarsus primus varus.

In common parlance, the term for hallux valgus is "bunion" (from the Greek for "turnip"), referring to the resulting prominence at the medial aspect of the first metatarsal head. A derivative term is **bunionette,** also once known as "tailor's bunion," describing a prominence lateral to the fifth metatarsal head, as in Figure 29.

So what's the varus or valgus relationship between the fifth metatarsal and the fifth proximal phalanx in bunionette? _____

Correct, if you answered varus, or digitus minimus varus (or digitus quintus varus, or digitus minimus pedis varus, or . . .).

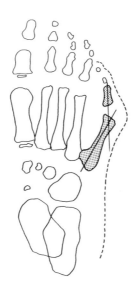

FIGURE 29. Bunionette.

Broken Midfoot

In general the above definitions of hindfoot and forefoot varus/valgus will usually result in an association of hindfoot valgus with forefoot valgus and hindfoot varus with forefoot varus. So why bother with evaluating both?

Well, in **broken midfoot,** there is *an uncoupling of the hindfoot from the forefoot.* Thus, the tight relationship of the calcaneus to all midfoot bones, and of the midfoot to the metatarsals is lost, at least to some extent. The broken midfoot may result from surgery, orthosis, or abnormal pressures (such as reversing right and left shoes to treat abnormal alignment). Broken midfoot has also been called Z-foot, referring to the abnormal fore-mid-hind-foot relationship as viewed from above or below. Thus, the configuration of hindfoot valgus with forefoot varus may be seen.

Metatarsus Adductus

In **metatarsus adductus** (L. *adducere* 'to draw toward'), toes are "turned in," i.e., *the forefoot deviates toward the midline.*

This is *not* a relationship between adjacent parts in series, as are varus and valgus; this is a positional statement about the toes (i.e., the metatarsals) themselves. Indeed, the most severe metatarsus adductus is associated with hindfoot valgus; Figure 30 shows such an association in a child whose toes turned in severely.

Please confirm by drawing the talar and calcaneal axis and calculating the angle (I get about 80°). Despite the metatarsus adductus, note that the formal forefoot relationship to the talus is also valgus.

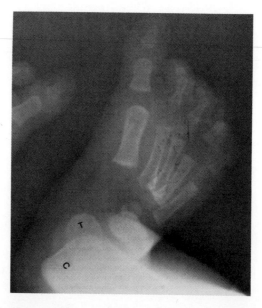

FIGURE 30. Metatarsus adductus with hindfoot valgus. (Reproduced, with permission, from Oestreich AE, Crawford AH. *Atlas of Pediatric Orthopedic Radiology.* Stuttgart: Thieme; 1985:259.)

4
Inversion, Eversion

Inversion   L. *in* "into" + *vertere* "to turn"
Eversion   L. *e* "out" + *vertere* "to turn"
inversion   rotation "inward" about the longitudinal axis of the foot
(i.e., great toe up, little toe down)
eversion   rotation "outward" about the longitudinal axis of the foot
(i.e., great toe down, little toe up)

Thus, it is the *sole* of the foot which goes in or out.

On frontal films, metatarsals and toes will overlap more than normal if the normal foot is inverted substantially.

It is in regard to forefoot varus/valgus and inversion/eversion that our approach and definitions differ from one traditional approach offered, for example, by Dr. Mike Ozonoff (*Pediatric Orthopedic Radiology*, 1979; Philadelphia: Saunders, pages 288–292). I try to fit forefoot valgus and varus into a universal definition of valgus and varus, as in Chapters 1 and 3 above; whereas the traditional approach cited above equates forefoot varus with inversion and forefoot valgus with eversion. In inversion (*traditional* forefoot varus), the bases of the metatarsals tend to converge more than normal and the proximal metatarsals are superimposed more than normal; while in eversion (*traditional* forefoot valgus), the metatarsals are less convergent than normal, more parallel, and with less overlap (see Figure 31).

Fortunately, most varus forefeet (according to my definition) are indeed inverted, including clubfeet at presentation, and there is also a tendency to eversion with most valgus forefeet (my definition), so that in general either method of varus/valgus definition can be used. Nevertheless, since varus and valgus at other sites refer to relationships between longitudinally adjacent parts, I contend that inversion/eversion ought to be considered separately from varus/valgus in the forefoot.

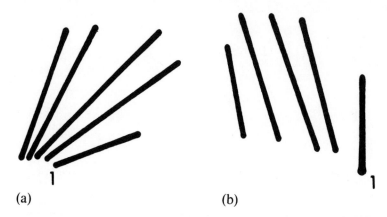

(a)   (b)

FIGURE 31. (a) Inverted left forefoot vs. (b) everted left forefoot. (Reproduced, with permission, from Ozonoff MB. *Pediatric Orthopedic Radiology.* Philadelphia: Saunders; 1979:289.)

On the lateral foot film, there is no potential for such disagreement or confusion. In inversion, the little toe becomes the lowest toe of 5 spread-out, relatively parallel toes, while in eversion, the great toe assumes the lowest position. (Invert or evert your foot to check this concept. No need to radiograph.)

Inversion is the same as foot **supination.**
Eversion is the same as foot **pronation.**

5
The Lateral Foot

On the lateral film it's important to consider the talo-calcaneal angle and its relation to hindfoot varus or valgus, cavus/planus, vertical/oblique talus, and the equinus or calcaneus calcaneus.

Let's begin with the normal talo-calcaneal angle on the weight-bearing or simulated weightbearing film. As on the frontal film, it is often easier to represent the calcaneus axis as a calcaneal margin which is easy to see—that means here the inferior calcaneal surface, although a midcalcaneus line can often be constructed. Usually one can esti-mate a midline talus axis fairly well (see Figure 32).

Although it isn't so far from the truth to remember 30° as the normal talo-calcaneal angle on the lateral film as well (as it is on the AP), it would be closer to choose 40°. Indeed, VanderWilde and colleagues re-port that through much of childhood there is a normal range of about 30–55° for this angle (see Figure 33).

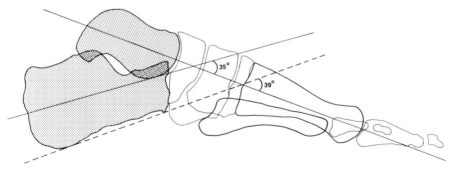

FIGURE 32. Calculating a talo-calcaneal angle, using midcalcaneal (solid) or lower calcaneal (dotted) line.

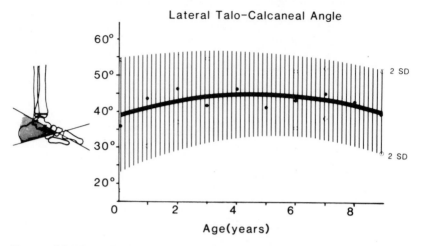

FIGURE 33. Normal range of the talo-calcaneal angle during childhood. (Reproduced, with permission, from VanderWilde R, Staheli LT, Chew DE, Magalon V. Measurements on radiographs of the foot in normal infants and children. *J Bone Jt Surg.* 1988;70A:407–415.)

This lateral talo-calcaneal angle does not directly measure varus or valgus. However, understanding the talo-calcaneal relationship in three dimensions (at least) allows preliminary opinions of hindfoot varus or valgus based on the weightbearing lateral film.

All other things being equal, let's look at the talus and calcaneus as a dynamic duo. Let your left hand represent the proximal (upper) bone, the talus, and your right hand represent the distal (lower) bone, the calcaneus. Keep your fingers (index-through-little finger) together and your hands flat.

Now let's "do" the AP talo-calcaneal angle of 0°: Place your flat left hand (facing to the right) directly on top of your flat right hand (facing to the left). Confirm from above the "talo-calcaneal angle" of 0°. Now lift your hands together (or tilt them) so that you can calculate the lateral "talo-calcaneal" angle.

You see, I hope, that the two hands' long axes are parallel, so that the angle here is also near 0°. Thus, when there is a varus talo-calcaneal relationship seen from above, there is associated a less-than-normal talo-calcaneal angle seen from the side.

Now, let's decrease the excessive support of the upper hand by the lower hand: that is, returning to your original position, rotate the lower hand approximately 30° about the wrist (the right hand moving, say, counterclockwise as viewed from above). Then the weight of the left fingers will allow them to descend somewhat, so that the lateral "talo-calcaneal angle" may now indeed be about 30–40°, the normal situation.

Finally, rotating the lower hand even more counterclockwise will deprive the "talus" of all "calcaneus" support, and it will tend to fall, fingers downward, into a position with even a greater "lateral talo-calcaneal angle."

So, if you have grasped the principles of this demonstration, you see that decreasing support of the talus by the calcaneus with increasing valgus is associated with an increasing lateral talo-calcaneal angle as well. And, when there is no major messing-up of tendons or other factors, it is true that a lower-than-normal talo-calcaneal angle on the weightbearing lateral film is characteristic of *varus;* and a greater-than-normal talocalcaneal angle on the lateral weightbearing film is characteristic of *valgus* between these two bones.

Cavus and Planus

In a **cavus** foot (i.e., *pes cavus,* from L. *cavus* 'hollow') the longitudinal arch is high.

In a **planus** foot (i.e., *pes planus,* from L. *planus* 'flat') the longitudinal arch is low to flat.

There are several ways for Measurers to evaluate the weightbearing lateral film for cavus or planus. The best way is probably just to decide by "eyeball" if the arch is high or low. The difference between weightbearing and non-weightbearing, incidentally, may be considerable. If the arch, instead of being flat is actually inverted (that is, *convex downward*), the term **rocker bottom foot** is used. The rocker-bottom may be the consequence, for example, of inadequate clubfoot treatment in which bony relationships have been weakened in an unbalanced fashion.

In the normal lateral weightbearing foot the midline axis of the talus fairly well runs through the midline axis of the first metatarsal. When the first metatarsal axis diverges anteriorly downward from the talus axis (i.e., the first metatarsal is significantly more steep in relationship to the horizontal), the cavus relationship is present (see Figure 34).

Alternatively, cavus may be judged by the angle between mid-calcaneus and first metatarsal axes. In this definition, either a more *calcaneus* position of the calcaneus (see below) *or* a steeper than normal descent of the first metatarsal, *or* both will mean cavus (see Figure 35).

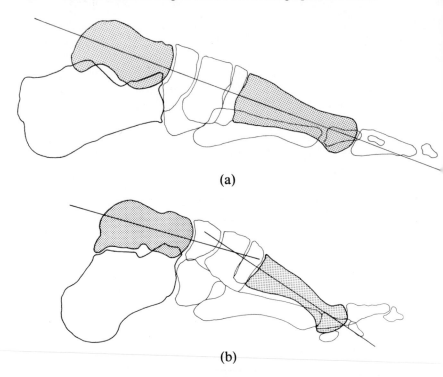

(a)

(b)

FIGURE 34. (a) Normal lateral weightbearing foot vs. (b) cavus foot.

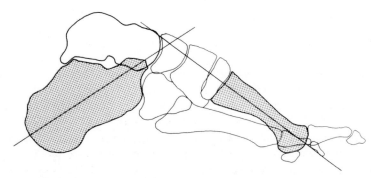

FIGURE 35. Alternate method for determining cavus.

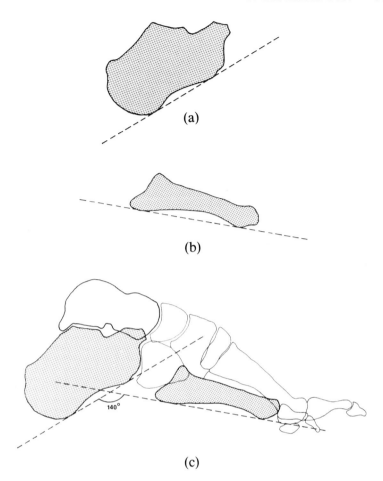

(a)

(b)

(c)

FIGURE 36. Third method for measuring cavus. In this method (a) a calcaneal line joins the outstanding lower points of the *calcaneus;* (b) a metatarsal line is based on the undersurface of the *fifth metatarsal.* (c) When the angle between the lines is less than about 150, cavus is present.

A third measuring method has been given in the useful article: Templeton AW, McAlister WH, Zim ID. Standardization of terminology and evaluation of osseous relationships in congenitally abnormal feet. *AJR.* 1965; 93: 374–381, as shown in Figure 36.

In this method, a calcaneal line joins the outstanding lower points of the *calcaneus* (see Figure 36a), while a metatarsal line is based on the undersuface of the *fifth metatarsal* (see Figure 36b). When the angle is less than about 150°, cavus is present (see Figure 36c).

Conversely, in planus, the talus axis may well extend downward compared to the first metatarsal axis; a decreased calcaneal-first metatarsal-midshaft angle will be seen; and the angle between the undersurfaces of the calcaneus and the fifth metatarsal will be increased (approaching 180°). An example allows you to observe the changes of planus (see Figure 37). (These changes should be even more marked in rocker-bottom foot.)

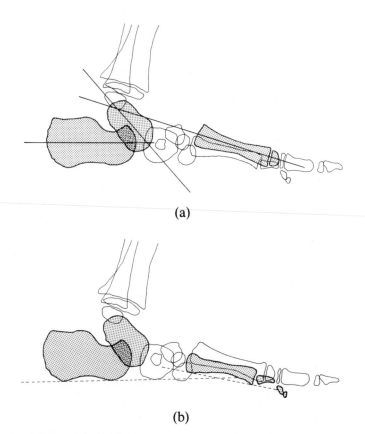

(a)

(b)

FIGURE 37. The planus foot, using the angles demonstrated in Figures 34–36.

Dr. Templeton and colleagues (*loc. cit.*) emphasize that in the child under five years of age, the central long axis of the talus on the lateral weightbearing film often normally passes inferior to the midshaft of the first metatarsal.

The Maximum Dorsiflexion Lateral

Especially in the evaluation of possible clubfoot and of treated known clubfoot, as well as tight heel cord, there is a value in considering the talo-calcaneal relationship on the **maximum dorsiflexion** lateral film. This title implies the attempt to dorsiflect the entire foot (i.e., undersurface of foot and ankle) with respect to the tibia. Although it is a few more pages until we define equinus, let me note here that the real use of this dorsiflexion film is to evaluate how much flexibility there is to an equinus position on the weightbearing lateral.

Once an adequate dorsiflexion view is obtained, the talo-calcaneal angle is measured by the same method as the weightbearing lateral. Again, we call upon Dr. VanderWilde's data to show that 40° is a good value to remember, although the very young child has values centering around 45° (see Figure 38).

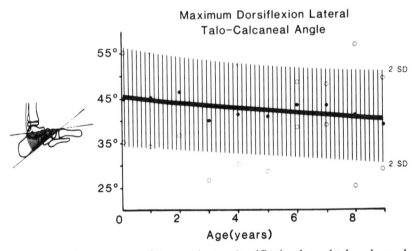

FIGURE 38. Normal range of the maximum dorsiflexion lateral talo-calcaneal angle in childhood. (Reproduced, with permission, from VanderWilde R, Staheli LT, Chew DE, Magalon V. Measurements on radiographs of the foot in normal infants and children. *J Bone Jt Surg.* 1988;70A:407–415.)

The Maximum Plantarflexion Lateral (Vertical Talus)

There is one situation in which it is essential to obtain the maximum plantarflexion lateral of a child's foot—that is, when there's a question of **vertical talus.**

In general, flat feet are valgus feet, and in general the lateral talocalcaneal angle is increased in valgus feet. In terms of surgical planning there is a major difference between vertical talus and the so-called oblique talus as the cause of a vertically appearing talus (very high talo-calcaneal angle) on the weightbearing lateral film.

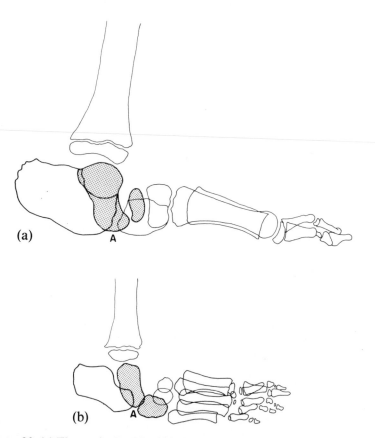

(a)

(b)

FIGURE 39. (a) The navicular (shaded) lies anterior to the dorsal surface of the talus, rather than to its anterior surface (point A). (b) In a younger child, the navicular is unossified, so we may evaluate the relative position of the cuboid (shaded) to the anterior surface (point A) of the talus.

In both true vertical and oblique talus, any ossified navicular appears to lie anterior to the dorsal (proximal) surface of the talus on the weightbearing lateral film. Which means you can't distinguish the two types of talus position abnormality by that criterion. If the navicular is not yet ossified but the cuboid is ossified (in the newborn, the cuboid probably isn't), then the cuboid may be a reasonable substitute for the navicular in evaluating talus position abnormality—i.e., the cuboid may lie anterior to the dorsal talar surface (Figure 39).

Even better, the unossified navicular, as well as its relationship to the talus, can be identified with ultrasound imaging, as demonstrated by Dr. A.E. Schlesinger at the 1989 meeting of the Society for Pediatric Radiology.

Now comes plantarflexion, which is important for this particular evaluation. On plantarflexion the true vertical talus shows a navicular (if ossified) still in front of the *dorsal* talus; while in oblique talus, which requires less extensive orthopedic treatment, the (ossified) navicular comes to lie in front of the *anterior* talus (Figure 40).

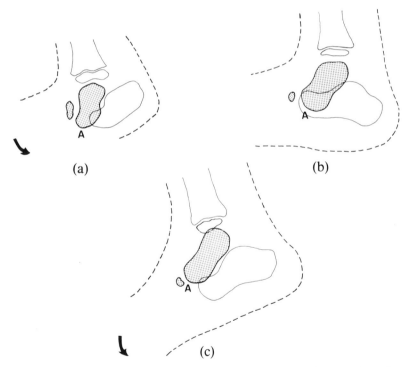

(a)

(b)

(c)

FIGURE 40. (a) Plantarflexion of true vertical talus. The navicular (shaded) remains in front of the dorsal talus. (b) Weightbearing view of oblique talus (simulates vertical talus). (c) Plantarflexion view of oblique talus. The navicular (shaded) comes to lie anterior to the anterior talus (point A).

Otherwise stated, in true vertical talus, the navicular remains well above the central talar axis despite plantarflexion.

In the young child without ossified navicular, on plantarflexion the cuboid is intersected by the talar central axis in oblique talus, while it (the cuboid) remains well above that line in vertical talus; or, if you prefer, in vertical talus on plantarflexion, the cuboid is still anterior to the dorsal talus, while in oblique talus the cuboid is anterior to the anterior talus.

Equinus and Calcaneus Calcaneus

We now arrive at the last major building blocks of basic foot evaluation, namely **equinus** (L. *equinus* 'relating to horses', from *equus* 'horse') and **calcaneus of the calcaneus.** (Yes, it is a bit strange that one of the two terms to describe abnormal calcaneus position is *calcaneus.*)

[L. *calcaneus* = calcaneus]

Let's get right to the mnemonics—then we'll discuss these relationships.

As seen in Figure 41, in the word "equinus," the lower case "q" at the front of the word extends downward below the rest of the lower case

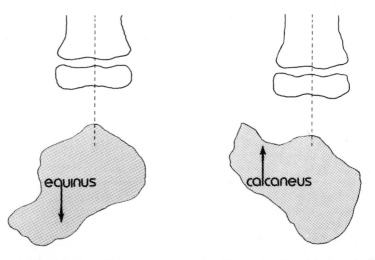

FIGURE 41. Equinus/calcaneus mnemonic. (Reproduced, with permission, from Oestreich AE, Crawford AH. *Atlas of Pediatric Orthopedic Radiology.* Stuttgart: Thieme; 1985:115.)

letters. In equinus position, the lower end of the calcaneus of the front of the bone extends relatively downward below the rest of the undersurface of the bone.

In "calcaneus," the lower case "l" at the front of the word extends upward above the rest of the lower case letters. In calcaneus position, the upper end of the calcaneus at the front of the bone extends relatively more upward than normal above the rest of the uppersurface of the bone.

On the weightbearing lateral film, calcaneus and equinus are used to express a relationship between the tibial central axis and the calcaneal bone (os calcis). So we want to look at the film as if we lined the tibia up in its normal anatomic position, i.e., vertically, and see where the calcaneus central axis (or undersurface axis) lies.

Normally the undersurface axis of the calcaneus is a bit higher anteriorly than posteriorly. Although in normal newborns, the calcaneus underface line may occasionally be perpendicular to the tibial axis, Dr. VanderWilde and colleagues report an anterior tibio-calcaneal angle mean of just over 75°, with that mean descending to near 65° at age 6, then increasing again slightly to age 9. (Please consult their article cited above if you require more numerical precision.) Otherwise, it's reasonable to describe equinus whenever the anterior calcaneus extends lower than the posterior, and when they are at the same level (i.e., 90° anterior tibio-calcaneal angle) beyond infancy. Calcaneus, being an abnormally tipped-up anterior calcaneus, as in many cavus feet, then means a low anterior tibio-calcaneal angle, especially 55° or below.

6
Clubfoot

At presentation, **clubfoot** is clinically obvious, and diagnosable without radiographs. The Diagnostic imaging would serve better to evaluate for congenital malformation syndromes, such as diastrophic dysplasia, that may foretell great difficulty in successful orthopedic treatment of clubfoot. Moreover, diagnostic imaging is pertinent for such associated conditions as tibial reduction deformity (viz., tibia hemimelia) or myelomeningocele.

When untreated clubfoot is radiographed, with weightbearing (or simulated weightbearing) AP and lateral films, plus maximal dorsiflexion lateral films, we should be able to apply all our skills developed so far in the course of this workbook:

The classic term for congenital clubfoot, is **talipes equinovarus**:

talipes (L. *talus* 'ankle' + *pes* 'foot') meant "ankle-foot," implying "walking on the ankle" and is used as a general term for a foot twisted out of shape. To some extent, this term reflects inversion of the foot present in clubfoot.

equinus is the disturbed relationship of calcaneus to tibia described in the last section.

varus includes hindfoot varus and forefoot varus, and, if you wish, inversion as well.

So let's mark up the example in Figure 42 and see what we get. (Littler bones are often harder to measure, aren't they?)

On the AP film the talus and calcaneus tend to overlap more fully than normal (i.e., angle near 0°)—which is hindfoot varus—and the first metatarsal lies medial to the central axis of the talus—which is forefoot varus by our definition. There may also be greater than normal convergence of the metatarsals proximally as well as overlap of their bases—the pattern of inversion.

On the weightbearing lateral, the talus and calcaneus tend to be parallel, i.e., lower than normal angle, a reflection of hindfoot varus, as

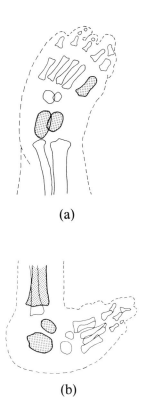

(a)

(b)

FIGURE 42. Talipes equinovarus.

discussed earlier. The calcaneus is indeed in equinus (tibio-calcaneal angle is _____). This parallelism and equinus persist on the maximum dorsiflexion lateral. Inversion is reflected by the inferiormost status of the fifth metatarsal, far from the uppermost first.

After treatment, the weightbearing and maximal dorsiflexion views may become completely normal in bony relationships; there may be residual or recurrent abnormalities resembling untreated clubfoot; there may be complications; and there are some secondary findings typical for treated clubfoot. An example of the latter would be the downward wedge-shape of the navicular on lateral films.

The radiographic findings do not always correlate with clinical results: a good clinical result may show incomplete normalization of relationships; clinical residual symptoms may accompany successful appearing x-rays.

A useful simple four-point approach is the following (Figure 43):

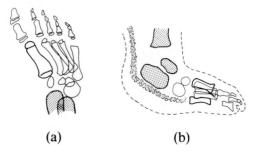

(a)   (b)

FIGURE 43. Example of a frontal (a) and lateral (b) foot after treatment for clubfoot, to be evaluated by the reader using the four-point approach described in the text.

1. Do the talus and calcaneus heads overlap on AP film? (If by much, it's still varus.)
2. Are the talus and calcaneus still parallel on the laterals? (If so, it's still varus.)
3. Is there still equinus? (If so, the heel cord is still too tight.)
4. Is there rocker-bottom foot? (Often a result of prolonged dorsiflexion without adequate addressing of equinus and hindfoot varus, this is a form of broken midfoot.)

Various other changes may also appear, beyond the scope of this workbook.

7
A Few Other Things

Tarsal Coalitions

The relationships between the bones of the feet and ankles are affected, naturally, when two or more usually separate bones are fused (whether the fusion is bony, cartilaginous, or fibrous). Symptoms are most likely to begin in the second decade, as ossification fills in the cartilaginous models of bone toward the definitive adult shape. Common symptoms of ankle bone coalitions are repeated sprains and strains, and, for some coalitions, painful pes planus (flat foot).

Most frequent among the tarsal coalitions is the calcaneonavicular bar, including bony, fibrous, and cartilaginous forms. Diagnosis is easy when the oblique view of the foot is obtained, which shows the close approach, or union, of the anteromedial corner of the calcaneus with the navicular. CT is not helpful for this diagnosis, and, indeed, may miss the coalition if only standard views are obtained. On the lateral foot or ankle film, the configuration of the anterosuperior corner of the calcaneus stretches into the appearance of an *anteater nose* which allows suspicion of talocalcaneal bar in situations in which the appropriate oblique has not yet been obtained (Figure 44).

(For more about the anteater nose, as well as the standard oblique view, please see Oestreich AE, Mize WA, Crawford AH, and Morgan RC: The "Anteater Nose": A Direct Sign of Calcaneonavicular Coalition on the Lateral Radiograph. *J Pediatr Orthop* 1987; 7:709–711. Thank you.)

The second most frequent tarsal coalition is the talo-calcaneal (or calcaneo-talar). This is a group of possible abnormal junction areas, most often lateral. It is often suspected incorrectly on lateral foot/ankle films, and often incorrectly unsuspected on lateral foot/ankle films. The frontal heel tomograms which can demonstrate these coalitions have been superceded by the far easier to perform CT exam. So for Calcaneo-Talar bars, CT is the way to go; while for Naviculo-Calcaneal bars, "No CT," but rather plain films, are the way.

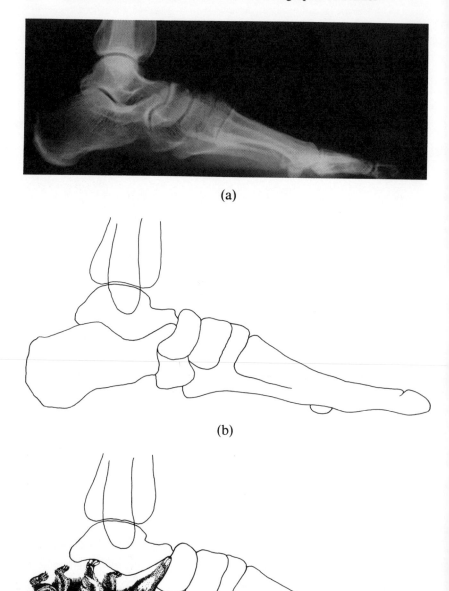

(a)

(b)

(c)

FIGURE 44. Anteater nose. (a) Radiograph. (b) Line drawing showing the long pointed anterior calcaneus. (c) Artist's view of anteater *qua* calcaneus.

The Ball-and-Socket Ankle

This refers to a convex, rather than flat, top to the talus on frontal views or frontal obliques; together with concave undersurface of the tibia and fibula that articulate with it (see Figure 45).

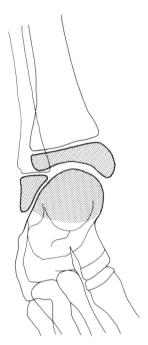

FIGURE 45. Ball-and-socket ankle (from a clinical example with only four toes).

Most of the time, there is an associated tarsal coalition. Most of the time, there is an associated deficiency in the number of toes. Often there are reduction deformities of the long bones of the ipsilateral lower extremity, including such deformities as absent fibula, short tibia, and proximal focal femoral deficiency. Typically, osseous maturation of the talus and its calcaneus are delayed. So discovery of the ball-in-socket ankle configuration should lead to full evaluation of that lower extremity.

The Accessory Navicular

The clinical **accessory navicular syndrome** comprises pain and a medially prominent accessory navicular bone, as for example in Figure 46.

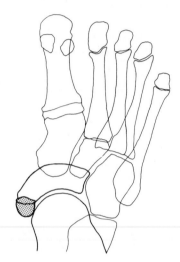

FIGURE 46. Accessory navicular (shaded).

As an "overuse" condition, there may be a need for corrective surgery, including reattachment of tendon to a new site, if conservative measures fail to cure symptoms. The same symptoms sometimes result from a medially prominent navicular without an accessory ossification.

The complex of navicular and accessory navicular therefore tend to have a varus relationship to the talus, yes?

Conclusion

By now you have mastered the basic concepts portrayed in this primer, and being "primed," you may proceed to your own clinical examples.

Best wishes

The Author

Index